Date: _____

Today's Verse:

_____
_____
_____
_____

Prayer:

_____
_____
_____
_____
_____

Today I am Thankful For:

_____
_____
_____
_____

Lord teach me to:

_____
_____
_____
_____

Date: _____

Today's Verse:

_____
_____
_____
_____

Prayer:

_____
_____
_____
_____
_____

Today I am Thankful For:

_____
_____
_____
_____

Lord teach me to:

_____
_____
_____
_____

Date: _____

Today's Verse:

_____
_____
_____
_____

Prayer:

_____
_____
_____
_____
_____

Today I am Thankful For:

_____
_____
_____
_____

Lord teach me to:

_____
_____
_____
_____

Date: _____

Today's Verse:

_____
_____
_____
_____

Prayer:

_____
_____
_____
_____
_____

Today I am Thankful For:

_____
_____
_____
_____

Lord teach me to:

_____
_____
_____
_____

Date: _____

Today's Verse:

_____
_____
_____
_____
_____

Prayer:

_____
_____
_____
_____
_____

Today I am Thankful For:

_____
_____
_____
_____

Lord teach me to:

_____
_____
_____
_____

Date: _____

Today's Verse:

_____
_____
_____
_____

Prayer:

_____
_____
_____
_____
_____

Today I am Thankful For:

_____
_____
_____
_____

Lord teach me to:

_____
_____
_____

Date: _____

Today's Verse:

_____
_____
_____
_____

Prayer:

_____
_____
_____
_____

Today I am Thankful For:

_____
_____
_____
_____

Lord teach me to:

_____
_____
_____
_____

Date: _____

Today's Verse:

_____
_____
_____
_____
_____

Prayer:

_____
_____
_____
_____
_____

Today I am Thankful For:

_____
_____
_____
_____

Lord teach me to:

_____
_____
_____
_____

Date: _____

Today's Verse:

_____
_____
_____
_____

Prayer:

_____
_____
_____
_____
_____

Today I am Thankful For:

_____
_____
_____
_____

Lord teach me to:

_____
_____
_____
_____

Date: _____

Today's Verse:

_____
_____
_____
_____

Prayer:

_____
_____
_____
_____

Today I am Thankful For:

_____
_____
_____
_____

Lord teach me to:

_____
_____
_____

Date: _____

Today's Verse:

_____
_____
_____
_____

Prayer:

_____
_____
_____
_____

Today I am Thankful For:

_____
_____
_____
_____

Lord teach me to:

_____
_____
_____

Date: _____

Today's Verse:

_____
_____
_____
_____
_____

Prayer:

_____
_____
_____
_____
_____

Today I am Thankful For:

_____
_____
_____
_____

Lord teach me to:

_____
_____
_____
_____

Date: _____

Today's Verse:

_____
_____
_____
_____

Prayer:

_____
_____
_____
_____

Today I am Thankful For:

_____
_____
_____
_____

Lord teach me to:

_____
_____
_____
_____

Date: _____

Today's Verse:

_____

_____

_____

_____

Prayer:

_____

_____

_____

_____

_____

Today I am Thankful For:

_____

_____

_____

_____

Lord teach me to:

_____

_____

_____

Date: _____

Today's Verse:

_____
_____
_____
_____
_____

Prayer:

_____
_____
_____
_____
_____

Today I am Thankful For:

_____
_____
_____
_____

Lord teach me to:

_____
_____
_____
_____

Date: _____

Today's Verse:

_____
_____
_____
_____

Prayer:

_____
_____
_____
_____
_____

Today I am Thankful For:

_____
_____
_____
_____

Lord teach me to:

_____
_____
_____
_____

Date: _____

Today's Verse:

_____
_____
_____
_____

Prayer:

_____
_____
_____
_____

Today I am Thankful For:

_____
_____
_____

Lord teach me to:

_____
_____
_____

Date: _____

Today's Verse:
_____
_____
_____
_____

Prayer:
_____
_____
_____
_____

Today I am Thankful For:
_____
_____
_____

Lord teach me to:
_____
_____
_____

Date: _____

Today's Verse:

_____
_____
_____
_____

Prayer:

_____
_____
_____
_____

Today I am Thankful For:

_____
_____
_____
_____

Lord teach me to:

_____
_____
_____

Date: _____

Today's Verse:

_____
_____
_____
_____

Prayer:

_____
_____
_____
_____
_____

Today I am Thankful For:

_____
_____
_____
_____

Lord teach me to:

_____
_____
_____
_____

Date: _____

Today's Verse:

_____
_____
_____
_____

Prayer:

_____
_____
_____
_____
_____

Today I am Thankful For:

_____
_____
_____

Lord teach me to:

_____
_____
_____

Date: _____

Today's Verse:

_____
_____
_____
_____

Prayer:

_____
_____
_____
_____

Today I am Thankful For:

_____
_____
_____
_____

Lord teach me to:

_____
_____
_____

Date: _____

Today's Verse:

_____
_____
_____
_____
_____

Prayer:

_____
_____
_____
_____
_____

Today I am Thankful For:

_____
_____
_____
_____

Lord teach me to:

_____
_____
_____
_____

Date: _____

Today's Verse:

_____
_____
_____
_____

Prayer:

_____
_____
_____
_____
_____

Today I am Thankful For:

_____
_____
_____
_____

Lord teach me to:

_____
_____
_____
_____

Date: _____

Today's Verse:

_____
_____
_____
_____
_____

Prayer:

_____
_____
_____
_____
_____

Today I am Thankful For:

_____
_____
_____
_____

Lord teach me to:

_____
_____
_____
_____

Date: _____

Today's Verse:

_____
_____
_____
_____
_____

Prayer:

_____
_____
_____
_____
_____

Today I am Thankful For:

_____
_____
_____
_____

Lord teach me to:

_____
_____
_____
_____

Date: _____

Today's Verse:

_____
_____
_____
_____

Prayer:

_____
_____
_____
_____
_____

Today I am Thankful For:

_____
_____
_____
_____

Lord teach me to:

_____
_____
_____
_____

Date: _____

Today's Verse:

_____
_____
_____
_____

Prayer:

_____
_____
_____
_____
_____

Today I am Thankful For:

_____
_____
_____
_____

Lord teach me to:

_____
_____
_____
_____

Date: _____

Today's Verse:

_____
_____
_____
_____

Prayer:

_____
_____
_____
_____

Today I am Thankful For:

_____
_____
_____
_____

Lord teach me to:

_____
_____
_____
_____

Date: _____

Today's Verse:

_____
_____
_____
_____

Prayer:

_____
_____
_____
_____
_____

Today I am Thankful For:

_____
_____
_____
_____

Lord teach me to:

_____
_____
_____
_____

Date: _____

Today's Verse:

_____
_____
_____
_____

Prayer:

_____
_____
_____
_____
_____

Today I am Thankful For:

_____
_____
_____
_____

Lord teach me to:

_____
_____
_____

Date: _____

Today's Verse:

_____
_____
_____
_____

Prayer:

_____
_____
_____
_____
_____

Today I am Thankful For:

_____
_____
_____
_____

Lord teach me to:

_____
_____
_____
_____

Date: _____

Today's Verse:

_____
_____
_____
_____

Prayer:

_____
_____
_____
_____

Today I am Thankful For:

_____
_____
_____
_____

Lord teach me to:

_____
_____
_____
_____

Date: _____

Today's Verse:

_____
_____
_____
_____

Prayer:

_____
_____
_____
_____
_____

Today I am Thankful For:

_____
_____
_____
_____

Lord teach me to:

_____
_____
_____
_____

Date: _____

Today's Verse:

_____
_____
_____
_____
_____

Prayer:

_____
_____
_____
_____
_____

Today I am Thankful For:

_____
_____
_____
_____

Lord teach me to:

_____
_____
_____
_____

Date: _____

Today's Verse:

_____
_____
_____
_____

Prayer:

_____
_____
_____
_____
_____

Today I am Thankful For:

_____
_____
_____
_____

Lord teach me to:

_____
_____
_____

Date: _____

Today's Verse:

_____
_____
_____
_____

Prayer:

_____
_____
_____
_____
_____

Today I am Thankful For:

_____
_____
_____
_____

Lord teach me to:

_____
_____
_____
_____

Date: _____

Today's Verse:

_____
_____
_____
_____
_____

Prayer:

_____
_____
_____
_____
_____

Today I am Thankful For:

_____
_____
_____
_____

Lord teach me to:

_____
_____
_____
_____

Date: _____

Today's Verse:

_____
_____
_____
_____

Prayer:

_____
_____
_____
_____

Today I am Thankful For:

_____
_____
_____
_____

Lord teach me to:

_____
_____
_____

Date: _____

Today's Verse:

_____
_____
_____
_____

Prayer:

_____
_____
_____
_____
_____

Today I am Thankful For:

_____
_____
_____
_____

Lord teach me to:

_____
_____
_____
_____

Date: _____

Today's Verse:

_____
_____
_____
_____

Prayer:

_____
_____
_____
_____

Today I am Thankful For:

_____
_____
_____
_____

Lord teach me to:

_____
_____
_____
_____

Date: _____

Today's Verse:

_____
_____
_____
_____

Prayer:

_____
_____
_____
_____
_____

Today I am Thankful For:

_____
_____
_____
_____

Lord teach me to:

_____
_____
_____
_____

Date: _____

Today's Verse:

_____
_____
_____
_____

Prayer:

_____
_____
_____
_____
_____

Today I am Thankful For:

_____
_____
_____
_____

Lord teach me to:

_____
_____
_____

Date: _____

Today's Verse:

_____
_____
_____
_____

Prayer:

_____
_____
_____
_____
_____

Today I am Thankful For:

_____
_____
_____

Lord teach me to:

_____
_____
_____

Date: _____

Today's Verse:

_____
_____
_____
_____

Prayer:

_____
_____
_____
_____

Today I am Thankful For:

_____
_____
_____

Lord teach me to:

_____
_____
_____

Date: _____

Today's Verse:

_____
_____
_____
_____

Prayer:

_____
_____
_____
_____

Today I am Thankful For:

_____
_____
_____
_____

Lord teach me to:

_____
_____
_____

Date: _____

Today's Verse:

_____
_____
_____
_____

Prayer:

_____
_____
_____
_____
_____

Today I am Thankful For:

_____
_____
_____
_____

Lord teach me to:

_____
_____
_____
_____

Date: _____

Today's Verse:

_____
_____
_____
_____

Prayer:

_____
_____
_____
_____
_____

Today I am Thankful For:

_____
_____
_____
_____

Lord teach me to:

_____
_____
_____
_____

Date: _____

Today's Verse:

_____
_____
_____
_____
_____

Prayer:

_____
_____
_____
_____
_____

Today I am Thankful For:

_____
_____
_____
_____

Lord teach me to:

_____
_____
_____
_____

Date: _____

Today's Verse:

_____
_____
_____
_____

Prayer:

_____
_____
_____
_____
_____

Today I am Thankful For:

_____
_____
_____
_____

Lord teach me to:

_____
_____
_____
_____

Date: _____

Today's Verse:

_____
_____
_____
_____
_____

Prayer:

_____
_____
_____
_____
_____

Today I am Thankful For:

_____
_____
_____
_____

Lord teach me to:

_____
_____
_____
_____

Date: _____

Today's Verse:

_____
_____
_____
_____

Prayer:

_____
_____
_____
_____

Today I am Thankful For:

_____
_____
_____

Lord teach me to:

_____
_____
_____

Date: _____

Today's Verse:

_____
_____
_____
_____

Prayer:

_____
_____
_____
_____
_____

Today I am Thankful For:

_____
_____
_____

Lord teach me to:

_____
_____
_____

Date: _____

Today's Verse:

_____
_____
_____
_____

Prayer:

_____
_____
_____
_____
_____

Today I am Thankful For:

_____
_____
_____
_____

Lord teach me to:

_____
_____
_____
_____

Date: _____

Today's Verse:

_____
_____
_____
_____

Prayer:

_____
_____
_____
_____

Today I am Thankful For:

_____
_____
_____
_____

Lord teach me to:

_____
_____
_____

Date: _____

Today's Verse:

_____
_____
_____
_____
_____

Prayer:

_____
_____
_____
_____
_____

Today I am Thankful For:

_____
_____
_____
_____

Lord teach me to:

_____
_____
_____
_____

Date: _____

Today's Verse:

_____
_____
_____
_____

Prayer:

_____
_____
_____
_____
_____

Today I am Thankful For:

_____
_____
_____
_____

Lord teach me to:

_____
_____
_____
_____

Date: _____

Today's Verse:

_____
_____
_____
_____

Prayer:

_____
_____
_____
_____

Today I am Thankful For:

_____
_____
_____
_____

Lord teach me to:

_____
_____
_____
_____

Date: _____

Today's Verse:

_____
_____
_____
_____

Prayer:

_____
_____
_____
_____

Today I am Thankful For:

_____
_____
_____
_____

Lord teach me to:

_____
_____
_____
_____

Date: _____

Today's Verse:

_____
_____
_____
_____

Prayer:

_____
_____
_____
_____
_____

Today I am Thankful For:

_____
_____
_____
_____

Lord teach me to:

_____
_____
_____
_____

Date: _____

Today's Verse:

_____
_____
_____
_____

Prayer:

_____
_____
_____
_____
_____

Today I am Thankful For:

_____
_____
_____
_____

Lord teach me to:

_____
_____
_____
_____

Date: _____

Today's Verse:

_____
_____
_____
_____
_____

Prayer:

_____
_____
_____
_____
_____

Today I am Thankful For:

_____
_____
_____
_____

Lord teach me to:

_____
_____
_____
_____

Date: _____

Today's Verse:

_____
_____
_____
_____
_____

Prayer:

_____
_____
_____
_____
_____

Today I am Thankful For:

_____
_____
_____
_____

Lord teach me to:

_____
_____
_____
_____

Date: _____

Today's Verse:

_____
_____
_____
_____

Prayer:

_____
_____
_____
_____
_____

Today I am Thankful For:

_____
_____
_____
_____

Lord teach me to:

_____
_____
_____
_____

Date: _____

Today's Verse:

_____
_____
_____
_____

Prayer:

_____
_____
_____
_____
_____

Today I am Thankful For:

_____
_____
_____
_____

Lord teach me to:

_____
_____
_____
_____

Date: _____

Today's Verse:

_____
_____
_____
_____

Prayer:

_____
_____
_____
_____
_____

Today I am Thankful For:

_____
_____
_____
_____

Lord teach me to:

_____
_____
_____
_____

Date: _____

Today's Verse:

_____
_____
_____
_____

Prayer:

_____
_____
_____
_____

Today I am Thankful For:

_____
_____
_____
_____

Lord teach me to:

_____
_____
_____
_____

Date: _____

Today's Verse:

_____
_____
_____
_____

Prayer:

_____
_____
_____
_____

Today I am Thankful For:

_____
_____
_____
_____

Lord teach me to:

_____
_____
_____
_____

Date: _____

Today's Verse:

_____
_____
_____
_____

Prayer:

_____
_____
_____
_____

Today I am Thankful For:

_____
_____
_____

Lord teach me to:

_____
_____
_____

Date: _____

Today's Verse:

_____
_____
_____
_____

Prayer:

_____
_____
_____
_____
_____

Today I am Thankful For:

_____
_____
_____
_____

Lord teach me to:

_____
_____
_____
_____

Date: _____

Today's Verse:

_____
_____
_____
_____

Prayer:

_____
_____
_____
_____
_____

Today I am Thankful For:

_____
_____
_____
_____

Lord teach me to:

_____
_____
_____
_____

Date: _____

Today's Verse:

_____
_____
_____
_____
_____

Prayer:

_____
_____
_____
_____
_____

Today I am Thankful For:

_____
_____
_____
_____

Lord teach me to:

_____
_____
_____
_____

Date: _____

Today's Verse:

_____
_____
_____
_____

Prayer:

_____
_____
_____
_____
_____

Today I am Thankful For:

_____
_____
_____
_____

Lord teach me to:

_____
_____
_____
_____

Date: _____

Today's Verse:

_____
_____
_____
_____

Prayer:

_____
_____
_____
_____
_____

Today I am Thankful For:

_____
_____
_____
_____

Lord teach me to:

_____
_____
_____
_____

Date: _____

Today's Verse:

_____
_____
_____
_____

Prayer:

_____
_____
_____
_____

Today I am Thankful For:

_____
_____
_____
_____

Lord teach me to:

_____
_____
_____

Date: _____

Today's Verse:

_____
_____
_____
_____
_____

Prayer:

_____
_____
_____
_____
_____

Today I am Thankful For:

_____
_____
_____
_____

Lord teach me to:

_____
_____
_____

Date: _____

Today's Verse:

_____
_____
_____
_____

Prayer:

_____
_____
_____
_____

Today I am Thankful For:

_____
_____
_____
_____

Lord teach me to:

_____
_____
_____

Date: _____

Today's Verse:

_____
_____
_____
_____

Prayer:

_____
_____
_____
_____
_____

Today I am Thankful For:

_____
_____
_____
_____

Lord teach me to:

_____
_____
_____
_____

Date: _____

Today's Verse:

_____
_____
_____
_____

Prayer:

_____
_____
_____
_____

Today I am Thankful For:

_____
_____
_____
_____

Lord teach me to:

_____
_____
_____

Date: _____

Today's Verse:

_____
_____
_____
_____

Prayer:

_____
_____
_____
_____
_____

Today I am Thankful For:

_____
_____
_____
_____

Lord teach me to:

_____
_____
_____
_____

Date: _____

Today's Verse:

_____
_____
_____
_____
_____

Prayer:

_____
_____
_____
_____
_____

Today I am Thankful For:

_____
_____
_____
_____

Lord teach me to:

_____
_____
_____
_____

Date: _____

Today's Verse:

_____
_____
_____
_____

Prayer:

_____
_____
_____
_____
_____

Today I am Thankful For:

_____
_____
_____
_____

Lord teach me to:

_____
_____
_____

Date: _____

Today's Verse:

_____
_____
_____
_____

Prayer:

_____
_____
_____
_____

Today I am Thankful For:

_____
_____
_____
_____

Lord teach me to:

_____
_____
_____

Date: _____

Today's Verse:

_____
_____
_____
_____

Prayer:

_____
_____
_____
_____
_____

Today I am Thankful For:

_____
_____
_____
_____

Lord teach me to:

_____
_____
_____
_____

Date: _____

Today's Verse:

_____
_____
_____
_____
_____

Prayer:

_____
_____
_____
_____
_____

Today I am Thankful For:

_____
_____
_____
_____

Lord teach me to:

_____
_____
_____
_____

Date: _____

Today's Verse:

_____
_____
_____
_____

Prayer:

_____
_____
_____
_____
_____

Today I am Thankful For:

_____
_____
_____
_____

Lord teach me to:

_____
_____
_____
_____

Date: _____

Today's Verse:

_____
_____
_____
_____

Prayer:

_____
_____
_____
_____

Today I am Thankful For:

_____
_____
_____
_____

Lord teach me to:

_____
_____
_____

Date: _____

Today's Verse:

_____
_____
_____
_____
_____

Prayer:

_____
_____
_____
_____
_____

Today I am Thankful For:

_____
_____
_____
_____

Lord teach me to:

_____
_____
_____

Date: _____

Today's Verse:

_____
_____
_____
_____
_____

Prayer:

_____
_____
_____
_____
_____

Today I am Thankful For:

_____
_____
_____
_____

Lord teach me to:

_____
_____
_____
_____

Date: _____

Today's Verse:

_____
_____
_____
_____

Prayer:

_____
_____
_____
_____
_____

Today I am Thankful For:

_____
_____
_____
_____

Lord teach me to:

_____
_____
_____

Date: _____

Today's Verse:

_____
_____
_____
_____

Prayer:

_____
_____
_____
_____
_____

Today I am Thankful For:

_____
_____
_____
_____

Lord teach me to:

_____
_____
_____
_____

Date: _____

Today's Verse:

_____
_____
_____
_____

Prayer:

_____
_____
_____
_____
_____

Today I am Thankful For:

_____
_____
_____
_____

Lord teach me to:

_____
_____
_____
_____

Date: _____

Today's Verse:

_____
_____
_____
_____

Prayer:

_____
_____
_____
_____

Today I am Thankful For:

_____
_____
_____

Lord teach me to:

_____
_____
_____

Date: _____

Today's Verse:

_____
_____
_____
_____

Prayer:

_____
_____
_____
_____
_____

Today I am Thankful For:

_____
_____
_____
_____

Lord teach me to:

_____
_____
_____
_____

Date: _____

Today's Verse:

_____
_____
_____
_____

Prayer:

_____
_____
_____
_____
_____

Today I am Thankful For:

_____
_____
_____
_____

Lord teach me to:

_____
_____
_____

Date: _____

Today's Verse:

_____
_____
_____
_____

Prayer:

_____
_____
_____
_____
_____

Today I am Thankful For:

_____
_____
_____
_____

Lord teach me to:

_____
_____
_____
_____

Date: _____

Today's Verse:

_____

_____

_____

_____

Prayer:

_____

_____

_____

_____

Today I am Thankful For:

_____

_____

_____

_____

Lord teach me to:

_____

_____

_____

_____

Date: _____

Today's Verse:

_____
_____
_____
_____

Prayer:

_____
_____
_____
_____
_____

Today I am Thankful For:

_____
_____
_____
_____

Lord teach me to:

_____
_____
_____

Date: _____

Today's Verse:

_____
_____
_____
_____

Prayer:

_____
_____
_____
_____

Today I am Thankful For:

_____
_____
_____

Lord teach me to:

_____
_____
_____

Date: _____

Today's Verse:

_____
_____
_____
_____

Prayer:

_____
_____
_____
_____

Today I am Thankful For:

_____
_____
_____
_____

Lord teach me to:

_____
_____
_____

Date: _____

Today's Verse:

_____
_____
_____
_____

Prayer:

_____
_____
_____
_____

Today I am Thankful For:

_____
_____
_____

Lord teach me to:

_____
_____
_____

Date: _____

Today's Verse:

_____
_____
_____
_____

Prayer:

_____
_____
_____
_____
_____

Today I am Thankful For:

_____
_____
_____
_____

Lord teach me to:

_____
_____
_____
_____

Date: _____

Today's Verse:

_____
_____
_____
_____

Prayer:

_____
_____
_____
_____

Today I am Thankful For:

_____
_____
_____
_____

Lord teach me to:

_____
_____
_____

Date: _____

Today's Verse:

_____
_____
_____
_____

Prayer:

_____
_____
_____
_____
_____

Today I am Thankful For:

_____
_____
_____
_____

Lord teach me to:

_____
_____
_____
_____

Date: _____

Today's Verse:

_____
_____
_____
_____

Prayer:

_____
_____
_____
_____
_____

Today I am Thankful For:

_____
_____
_____
_____

Lord teach me to:

_____
_____
_____
_____

Date: _____

Today's Verse:

_____
_____
_____
_____
_____

Prayer:

_____
_____
_____
_____
_____

Today I am Thankful For:

_____
_____
_____
_____

Lord teach me to:

_____
_____
_____
_____

Date: _____

Today's Verse:

_____
_____
_____
_____

Prayer:

_____
_____
_____
_____

Today I am Thankful For:

_____
_____
_____
_____

Lord teach me to:

_____
_____
_____
_____

Date: _____

Today's Verse:

_____
_____
_____
_____

Prayer:

_____
_____
_____
_____
_____

Today I am Thankful For:

_____
_____
_____
_____

Lord teach me to:

_____
_____
_____
_____

Date: _____

Today's Verse:

_____
_____
_____
_____

Prayer:

_____
_____
_____
_____
_____

Today I am Thankful For:

_____
_____
_____
_____

Lord teach me to:

_____
_____
_____
_____

Date: _____

Today's Verse:

_____
_____
_____
_____

Prayer:

_____
_____
_____
_____
_____

Today I am Thankful For:

_____
_____
_____
_____

Lord teach me to:

_____
_____
_____

Date: _____

Today's Verse:

_____
_____
_____
_____

Prayer:

_____
_____
_____
_____

Today I am Thankful For:

_____
_____
_____
_____

Lord teach me to:

_____
_____
_____

Date: _____

Today's Verse:

_____
_____
_____
_____

Prayer:

_____
_____
_____
_____

Today I am Thankful For:

_____
_____
_____

Lord teach me to:

_____
_____
_____

Date: _____

Today's Verse:

_____
_____
_____
_____

Prayer:

_____
_____
_____
_____
_____

Today I am Thankful For:

_____
_____
_____
_____

Lord teach me to:

_____
_____
_____

Date: _____

Today's Verse:

_____
_____
_____
_____

Prayer:

_____
_____
_____
_____
_____

Today I am Thankful For:

_____
_____
_____
_____

Lord teach me to:

_____
_____
_____
_____

Date: _____

Today's Verse:

_____
_____
_____
_____

Prayer:

_____
_____
_____
_____
_____

Today I am Thankful For:

_____
_____
_____
_____

Lord teach me to:

_____
_____
_____

Date: _____

Today's Verse:

_____
_____
_____
_____
_____

Prayer:

_____
_____
_____
_____
_____

Today I am Thankful For:

_____
_____
_____
_____

Lord teach me to:

_____
_____
_____

Date: _____

Today's Verse:

_____
_____
_____
_____

Prayer:

_____
_____
_____
_____

Today I am Thankful For:

_____
_____
_____
_____

Lord teach me to:

_____
_____
_____

Date: _____

Today's Verse:

_____
_____
_____
_____

Prayer:

_____
_____
_____
_____

Today I am Thankful For:

_____
_____
_____
_____

Lord teach me to:

_____
_____
_____

Date: _____

Today's Verse:

_____
_____
_____
_____

Prayer:

_____
_____
_____
_____

Today I am Thankful For:

_____
_____
_____
_____

Lord teach me to:

_____
_____
_____

Date: _____

Today's Verse:

_____
_____
_____
_____

Prayer:

_____
_____
_____
_____
_____

Today I am Thankful For:

_____
_____
_____
_____

Lord teach me to:

_____
_____
_____
_____

Date: _____

Today's Verse:

_____
_____
_____
_____

Prayer:

_____
_____
_____
_____

Today I am Thankful For:

_____
_____
_____

Lord teach me to:

_____
_____
_____

Date: _____

Today's Verse:

_____
_____
_____
_____

Prayer:

_____
_____
_____
_____

Today I am Thankful For:

_____
_____
_____
_____

Lord teach me to:

_____
_____
_____